PROGRAMME

by
Dr Amanda Roberts
M.B. B.Chir

KENNETH MASON
EMSWORTH

THIS IS NOT *YET ANOTHER DIET* –

It is a programme designed to help you achieve and maintain your optimum shape. This programme is a four week low fat diet combined with gentle exercises specifically chosen to ensure that fat is lost from those problem areas; hips, thighs, stomach, upper arms and chin.

We conclude with suggestions for your maintenance plan. Any diet can tell you what to eat for a short period of time but a successful diet needs to ensure you don't gain those extra bulges again. The guidelines in this book help you organise your own maintenance programme: you can adapt the diet to suit your own tastes and lifestyle.

Why this programme works!

• It has been designed to be very easy to follow.

• The diet foods are quick to prepare and appetising for the whole family.

• It educates and informs you about the *danger* foods, those very fattening foods to definitely avoid.

• It guides you to the foods that will help you achieve the shape you desire.

• It teaches you that you are *not* punishing

2

yourself by *'going on a diet'*. You are simply learning about the content of the foods you eat or want to eat, essential if you really want to lose weight.

• It helps you try new less fattening ways of preparing food and possibly sample completely new foods.

• It is designed to be highly enjoyable.

Why you should try this programme

Not only to lose weight and gain a better shape but also to improve your health, to reduce your risk of heart disease and other problems caused by or aggravated by obesity.

In 1990 the government published a study of British eating habits; it is a survey of one weeks food and drink intake by two thousand people. It showed that three times as many women are overweight now than were six years ago. The number of men overweight had risen by one third. It has long been recommended that less than one third of our diet comes from fat but on the whole we eat more fat than ever and most of it is saturated fat – believed to be the most harmful sort.

Reasons why many of us find it hard to control our weight

1. Too much saturated fat
80% of us eat too much saturated fat in popular foods like milk, eggs, ham, cheese, chips and meat.

2. Too many sweet things
Cakes and biscuits and chocolates all have high sugar and fat content.

3. Not enough fibre
The recommended daily allowance of fibre is 30 g. It is found in bread, potatoes, lentils and cereals. While dieting fibre provides bulk without calories and thus reduces hunger pangs.

4. Not enough exercise
Most of our day to day manual tasks have been made easier by machines – dishwashers, electric lawnmowers etc. We don't even have to move to change TV channels.

5. We eat out more
Eating out has become more popular, making it harder to control what you eat.

6. Too much alcohol
Alcohol is very much part of our lives now. It is important for health and figure to watch our intake and be aware of higher calorie drinks.

Understanding diets

Crash diets DO NOT WORK. They may reduce your weight but rarely improve your figure; the weight loss is seldom lasting. It is important to understand why many diets do not work, why they make us listless, irritable and sometimes even depressed. Severe diets are hard to stick to. They encourage binging and cheating. If you feel a diet is punishing you it is only too easy to stray and reward yourself with forbidden foods. The fat we want to lose needs energy to mobilise from the body stores and convert itself into energy. Crash diets do not provide this energy. Our brains need glucose; if it is not present in our diet we will break down muscle (*protein*) in preference to fat to provide glucose. We may lose weight but it will not be fat weight. Without proper attention to the correct balance of meals, high protein and low calorie diets can lead to dizziness, bad temper and cravings for carbohydrates, e.g. sugary, starchy foods.

> **We need a balanced diet at all times – even when dieting**

This programme concentrates on shape rather than weight. There is no goal to lose x number of pounds or kilos a week. The aim is to achieve and maintain a shape you are happy with. I include a weight chart mainly as a preliminary check. *You should not* start this or any other diet without a medical check first. If you are in the overweight section of the weight chart you should probably lose weight but remember with this or any other diet please check with your doctor first. Never aim to weigh less than the lowest recommended weight for your height.

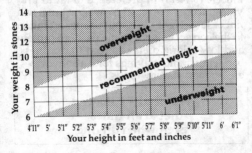

Nutritional requirements

- **Protein** found in meat, eggs, dairy products, pulses and vegetables. 11% of our daily calorie intake should be protein.
- **Carbohydrates** are sugars and starches. They should provide between 50% and 70% of our calorie requirements. Sugars are found in brown & white sugar as well as fruit, and starches in beans, grain and rice.
- **Fibre** is indigestible carbohydrate found in plant material, it is very important for healthy bowels. While dieting it provides bulk and staves off hunger pangs without increasing calories.
- **Fats** fall into three main groups:

Saturated in meat and dairy products.

Monounsaturated in olive oil and avocados.

Polyunsaturated in fish and vegetable oils. Less than 30% of our calories should come from fats.

We eat too much saturated fats

Many people not clinically overweight do not look or feel fit ... Many of us have little energy, bad posture, bulging tummies, sagging bustlines, flabby upper arms and more than one chin. You can improve on all these with attention to diet, a small amount of exercise, and correction of bad posture rather than frantic crash dieting and loss of weight. Dieting again and again does not work to control our shape ... only altering our diet does.

Most of us eat far more than we need and there is no doubt that we all eat too much fat. In the western world the average daily fat intake is 120 g: we need less than 30 g. Some people burn this excess fat off easily, the less fortunate of us store it on our hips, thighs and tummies. To achieve our ideal shape we must regulate our fat intake and take a moderate amount of exercise.

Below are calorie values of food groups, to show how fat and alcohol contribute to the calories we eat.

1g protein	=	4 Kcal	17Kj
1g carbohydrate	=	3.75 Kcal	16Kj
1g fat	=	9 Kcal	37Kj
1g alcohol	=	7 Kcal	29Kj

Fat contains over double the calories of other food groups. It is essential to have some fat in the diet. The number of calories present depends on the total content of the different types of fat. Research into general health has shown that a diet low in saturated fats is healthier and that unsaturated fats such as are found in fish oils may help prevent heart disease. Alcohol has almost double the calories of foods other than fats but unfortunately has no nutritional value at all.

Cholesterol is present in certain foods and is a product of fat metabolism. High blood cholesterol often accompanies cardiovascular disease. Cholesterol is a vital raw material for making certain body hormones and bile salts; only when levels of cholesterol in the blood are too high is it considered unhealthy.

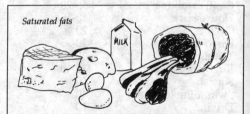

Saturated fats

Understanding our fat & calorie intake

The DHSS report on *diet and cardiovascular disease* recommends everyone reduce their fat intake by one third.

They also recommend a calorie intake of 1,800 - 2,100 calories per day for women and 2,300 - 2,600 for men. The older you get after the age of eighteen the less calories you need. Young teenagers need the highest intake of calories for healthy development.

Our calorie requirements vary depending on age and occupation. This table gives an idea of the calories used for various activities. Judge yourself if your calorie needs are high or low and whether you should have large or small portions. Men almost always need larger portions.

	Kcals/5 mins
Office work	7-10
Gentle walking	15-20
Housework	10-15
Cycling	20
Disco dancing	30-35
Tennis	25-30
Rugby or Soccer	30-40
Squash	60
Swimming lengths	40
Driving	10

Where does all the fat come from?

These figures compare the different amounts of fat in various food. We eat a great deal of fat without realising it. The figures may surprise you. Take note of them, and ask yourself – how much is in my favourite food? Could I change to a similar low fat alternative?

In one pint of milk

	Full cream
Fat	23g
Protein	19g
Carbohydrate	27g
Total energy	385Kcal

	Semi-skimmed
Fat	10g
Protein	19g
Carbohydrate	28g
Total energy	275Kcal

	Skimmed
Fat	1g
Protein	19g
Carbohydrate	28g
Total energy	195Kcal

Get to know high and low fat contents

		g per 100g
Oils, cooking and salad		100
Butter and margarine		81
Low fat spreads		40
Lean rumpsteak grilled		6
Beefburger grilled		24
Pork pie		28
Chicken roast	with skin	14
	no skin	5
Yoghurt,	greek style	10
	very low fat	0.1
Cream,	clotted	60
	low fat	8.6
Cheese,	cottage	1.5
	cheddar	34
Quiche		16
Biscuits,	cream crackers	14
	water biscuits	7
Eggs boiled		10

These are the fundamental ideas on which *The Hip & Thigh Programme* is based

- Eat less fat

- Eat less calories *mainly by reducing your fat intake*

- Balance your diet from all four food groups

- Drink plenty of fluids
  see page 27 drinks

- Learn to substitute similar foodstuffs to vary your diet and to make it more interesting.

- Take an interest in what you are eating. Is there fat in it? Is there fibre in it? Are there a lot of calories in it?

- Gentle exercises to tone up the muscles crucial to looking and feeling good.

Tips on changing fattening habits

1. *Do not drink whole milk.* Avoid dishes or sauces which contain full fat cream.

2. *Reduce sugar in drinks.* Use artificial sweeteners. Cans of fizzy drink contain the equivalent of 10 lumps of sugar each, select **diet, low cal or lite** versions.

3. *Do not snack.* Eat three meals a day.

4. *Do not skip meals.* You will get hungry at inconvenient times and fill up on fatty snacks or fast foods.

5. *Save cakes and biscuits* for birthdays and holidays. If you really love them it is worth waiting: you may not miss them.

6. *Be aware* of how food is prepared. Grill and cook in the oven. Cook in stock, wine or cider instead of oil and fat.

7. *Avoid fast foods.* Hamburgers, hotdogs, chips, doughnuts are all disasters. The sizzling burger on the cinema screen looks good, but the limp fatty bun and meat you buy in the foyer is always bad for you.

8. Use low fat spreads not butter. Low fat yoghurts and creme fraiche instead of cream in recipes. Try half fat cream.

9. Buy and eat more vegetables.

10. Try different breads. If you hate brown bread try high fibre white. Avoid rubbery white sliced bread.

11. Eat more potatoes. Cottage cheese or low fat fromage frais is tasty with jacket potatoes instead of butter. Avoid fried potatoes.

12. Reduce your alcohol consumption.

13. Do not eat chicken skin or any of the fat visible on meat.

14. Eat only three to four eggs a week.

15. Walk more. Use stairs not lifts where practical.

16. No second helpings.

17. Choose fresh fruit or fruit salad as a dessert in restaurants. Avoid cheese.

How determined are you to shape up?

• You must look forward to the next four weeks and not dread them.

• Familiarise yourself with the menus, try out a few dishes before starting in earnest.

• Make a definite time in the day for your exercises.

• Remember this is not just a diet: you are learning all about what you must eat in order to maintain a figure you are happy with.

• For a week before you start the diet get used to eating three meals a day, avoiding between meal snacks, and cutting down on alcohol. Drink more water.

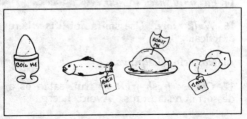

The following foods are not part of the diet and *should not* be eaten in the first four weeks.

No butter, margarine or margarine substitutes except where indicated in the recipes.

No whole milk, cream or milk products, puddings, ice cream, yoghurts, creamy sauces etc.

No crisps or nuts.

No sweets, chocolate or chocolate & cocoa products.

No sweet or savoury biscuits except water biscuits and ryvita.

No oily salad dressings or mayonnaise.

No oily fish *(can be eaten in maintenance diet).*

No foods cooked or basted in oil.

No prepared meat products i.e. sausages, luncheonmeat, pork pies, pate etc.

No fast foods.

No chips.

The diet

There is an old saying that we should eat breakfast like a king, lunch like a prince and supper like a pauper. Few of us allow for proper breakfast or lunch and for social reasons tend to have our main meal with family and friends in the evenings.

As long as you have one breakfast, light meal and main meal you will be following the diet. If you can have a larger breakfast eat two specified breakfasts together, then have one light meal and one main course only main meal, with plenty of vegetables.

Have at least one protein containing meal per day. If you are still hungry after the light meal eat a piece of fresh fruit. I have shown three courses for the main meal, you don't have to eat all three. You may eat unlimited vegetables, fruit, potato, rice or egg free pasta. Be reasonable and don't add butter.

Diet plan for ten days

You may follow this or make your own menus exchanging similar meals. I have made a ten day plan which you can repeat three times or follow for ten days and then substitute your own plan. The idea of this programme is that you learn to plan your day to day food intake.

I recommend starting this diet on a Monday so that the larger meals and those which take more time to prepare will fall at the weekend. Start on a Monday and you can shop at the weekend for the foods you'll need for your new regime.

Day 1

B Choice of cereal
L Baked potato with coleslaw
D Melon
  Grilled fish, peas, carrots and rice
  Baked apple

Day 2

B Fresh fruit salad
L Cottage cheese sandwich
D Carrot soup
  Chicken in the pot
  Sorbet

Day 3
B Low fat fruit yoghurt
L Tuna and bean salad
D Tomato soup
Shepherds pie
Baked bananas

Day 4
B Baked beans on toast
L Turkey and celery sandwich
D Cucumber in yoghurt
Pasta with tuna
Tropical fruit salad

Day 5
B Choice of cereal
L Baked potato with cottage cheese
D Tomatoes with basil
Fish pie
Pears with blueberries

Day 6
B Tomatoes and mushrooms on toast
L Stir fry with rice
D Crudites
Chicken in cider
Pavlova

Day 7

B Poached egg on toast with tomatoes
L Chicken breast with watercress salad
D Mushrooms with garlic
Poached salmon
Summer pudding

Day 8

B Low fat yoghurt
L Tomato and cucumber sandwich
D Soup
Roast chicken
Oranges with toffee

Day 9

B Choice of cereal
L Baked potato with ratatouille
D Grated carrot
Chilli con carne
Tropical fruit salad

Day 10

B Boiled egg with toast
L Pasta with tuna
D Soup
Ratatouille with rice
Apricot flan

You will see that days 1 & 8 are especially light: you should start the diet plan on a Monday as we often eat and drink more at weekends and this compensates for the increased intake. Keep Monday as a light day during your maintenance plan.

You can swap dishes that you do not like or are not convenient for others from the same list. Try to exchange a dish for one similar in carbohydrate, protein or fibre.

You can have your main meal at lunch time or at breakfast provided your other two meals are light.

Light breakfasts
Don't forget your glass of water.
1 cup of tea or coffee
Unsweetened juice
with either
1 piece of toast with one of:
- fresh fruit salad
- exotic fruit – mango, pawpaw or melon
- very low fat fruit yoghurt
- tinned fruit in juice
- diced apple & banana in lemon juice
- mashed banana with low fat yoghurt

or

25 g serving of unsweetened cereal
- puffed or shredded wheat
- bran flakes or cornflakes
- puffed rice or muesli without nuts

These may be served with skimmed milk or fruit juice. Muesli soaked in fruit juice is delicious. Add fresh fruit to cereals as a way of sweetening them.

Cooked breakfasts

Tomatoes & mushrooms on toast 2 tomatoes chopped with 50 g mushrooms. Cook together in a non-stick pan slowly and pour over one slice of wholemeal toast.

Poached egg with tomato serve together on brown toast

Baked beans on toast 1 slice toast and 225 g low sugar beans.

Boiled egg with two slices of toast.

Porridge made with skimmed milk and sweetened with one teaspoon brown sugar.

If breakfast is to be your main meal eat one cooked and one light and increase the size of portion

Light meals

May be eaten for lunch or dinner or both if you are having a large breakfast.

Pasta with tuna or tomatoes *hot or cold*.

Baked potato with baked beans, add mustard to the beans.

Baked potato with cottage cheese. Chives or pineapple liven this up.

Baked potato with coleslaw made with low fat yoghurt, lemon juice black pepper.

Sandwiches

- Marmite and fresh mint
- Chicken, tomato and salad
- Tuna and lettuce *(tuna in brine not oil)*
- Grated carrot with orange pieces
- Cottage cheese *(low fat)* with herbs
- Turkey breast with celery
- Mashed banana

Use only low fat spread or no spread and some low fat yoghurt to moisten the filling.

Stir fry with rice

Leek and potato soup

Chicken and salad skinned, grilled chicken breast with watercress salad and boiled new potatoes rolled in low fat yoghurt and fresh parsley.

...ey breast and salad 2 slices with red
...bage and orange salad served with a small
baked potato.

Tuna salad either tuna salad with beans
(page 32) or tuna in brine mixed with low fat
yoghurt served on bed of shredded lettuce.

Ratatouille and rice

Dinners

Most of us do not eat a three course dinner
everyday. You need the variety of foods so
eat smaller portions rather than cut out
courses. Vegetables and fresh fruits are important in the diet, if you are hungry you
should eat more of these.

Hors d'oevres/first course

Mushrooms, fresh garlic & parsley
Italian bean and tuna salad
Soups: tomato, carrot, minestrone, gazpacho
Stuffed tomatoes or red peppers
Grated carrot with small pieces of
orange.
Cucumber in yoghurt peeled and thinly
sliced cucumber in plain low fat yoghurt

with black pepper and lots of garlic.

Tomatoes with fresh basil add crushed garlic, chopped fresh basil and black pepper to sliced ripe tomatoes. Leave in the fridge for an hour before eating.

Cruditee grated carrot, beetroot, celeriac with sliced cucumber.

Melon serve plain, with ginger or black pepper.

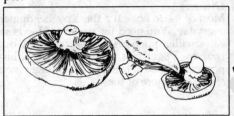

Main courses

Ratatouille
Leek & potato soup with or without mussels cooked in cider
Chicken in the pot, cooked in cider, roast.
Grilled fish
Poached salmon
Fish pie

...ana or tomato and fresh basil
...n rump steak (150g)

Desserts

Apricot & cherry flan
Baked bananas with brown sugar
Green fruit salad
Baked apple
Tropical fruit salad with passion fruit
Tania's pavlova
Oranges with toffee
Sorbet mango and passion fruit, raspberry
Ice cream blackberry, raspberry
Pears with blueberries
Low fat rice pudding

Drinks

We drink far less fluid than we should and
too great a percentage of our fluid intake is
made up of tea, coffee and alcohol. Limit
cups of tea and coffee to 2 or 3 cups a day,
drink more fruit juice, water and herbal teas.
While on the diet drink 250 ml skimmed milk

a day in tea, coffee or
allowed but no more th
for females and 8 units for i
is a glass of wine, a single meas
or half a pint of beer. On the diet t
only dry white wine: if you drink spi
should be neat, with water or low calc
mixes.

Above all drink more water

Recipes

Pasta with tuna   *serves 4*

120 g egg free pasta
200 g tin of tuna in brine
1 small onion
1 teaspoon olive oil
380 g tin peeled plum tomatoes
1 teaspoon of turmeric *(optional)*

Boil pasta in plenty of water. Put water on to
boil while you make the sauce, heat olive oil
in a thick bottomed pan. Add the onion and
stir on a low heat until the onion softens.
Add the tuna and the tomatoes. Drain the
juice unless you like your sauce runny. Add

the turmeric and cook on a low heat for 10 minutes. Pour sauce over pasta and serve piping hot.

Pasta with basil & tomatoes   *serves 4*
120 g egg free pasta
4 large tomatoes or 380 g tin peeled plum tomatoes *ripe fresh tomatoes are best if you want to eat this cold.*
4 dessert spoons finely chopped fresh basil
1 teaspoon olive oil
Fresh garlic, crushed or finely chopped
Boil pasta in plenty of water. Finely chop tomatoes, put in pan after the olive oil and garlic. Heat through and pour over the pasta. Mix together with fresh basil.

Ratatouille   *serves 4*
2 large aubergines *(eggplant)*
4 courgettes
1 large onion, chopped
2 cloves garlic crushed *(optional)*
2 380 g tins plum tomatoes *(drain juice)*
2 bay leaves
1 teaspoon oil
1 glass of dry white wine
This is very good cooked in a slow cooker. First heat oil in a deep pan, then add onion

and garlic. Chop aubergines into small squares. Slice courgettes in thick slices. Add the wine, aubergines and courgettes, then tomatoes, bay leaves, some freshly milled black pepper and a little salt. Add water to nearly cover. Cook slowly until the aubergines are soft. You can cook it faster but you need to stir often and the vegetables tend to break up. Serve hot with rice or baked potato, or alone as a first course.

Stir fry with rice
serves 4

12 oz diced chicken breast or monkfish marinated for at least an hour in 2 tablespoons soy sauce.
Juice of half a lemon
1 tablespoon white wine vinegar
6 oz shredded white cabbage
12 oz beansprouts, fresh
6 oz sliced button mushrooms
1 teaspoon oil, half cup of vegetable stock
In a large pan or wok boil the cabbage in the stock until it evaporates. Then add oil, mushrooms and chicken or monkfish. Stir fry until meat or fish is cooked, 2-3 mins, and add the beansprouts. Add salt and black pepper. Serve with brown or white rice.

lid on and sweat over a low heat. Stir a couple of times until the leeks are soft, about 5 minutes. Add the orange juice and water. Boil for 10 minutes. When cool liquidise half, return to pan, reheat and serve. Add parsley just before serving.

Tomato soup
serves 6

2 large tins peeled plum tomatoes
750 ml chicken or vegetable stock
1 small onion finely chopped
freshly milled black pepper
1 teaspoon of brown sugar
1 tablespoon chopped fresh parsley or basil

Cook onion in a little stock until soft. Finely chop tomatoes, add pepper and sugar with the rest of the stock. Bring to the boil. Liquidise and add the parsley or basil.

Minestrone
serves 4

This soup can be a light meal it you replace pasta with a tin of drained kidney beans.

1 small onion, finely chopped
1 clove garlic, crushed
1 teaspoon olive oil
380 g tin peeled plum tomatoes, chopped
2 sticks celery finely chopped
half teaspoon dried oregano

1 bayleaf, pinch dried rosemary
2 teaspoons fresh basil
2 tablespoons tomato concentrate
salt and freshly milled black pepper
2 medium carrots and half a green pepper
finely diced
850 ml vegetable stock
25 g vermicelli
1 tablespoon chopped fresh parsley

Put oil, onion, celery and garlic in bottom of
thick pan. Cover and sweat over a low heat
for 5 minutes. Then add other ingredients
except vermicelli and parsley. Simmer for
half an hour then add the vermicelli, simmer
until cooked. Add parsley just before serving.

Gazpacho

serves 4

560 g ripe tomatoes, finely chopped
2 spring onions, finely chopped
quarter cucumber, finely chopped
2 cloves garlic, crushed
1 small green pepper
1 heaped tablespoon chopped fresh basil
1 heaped tablespoon chopped fresh parsley
half tablespoon chopped chives
half tablespoon chopped fresh marjoram
3 tablespoons wine vinegar

freshly milled black pepper
tabasco sauce and salt to taste
300 ml tomato juice
3 slices wholemeal bread, finely crumbled
Mix all the ingredients together and keep in the fridge stirring occasionally. This soup must be served icy cold so make at least three hours before eating.

Stuffed red peppers
serves 4

4 red peppers
1 teaspoon olive oil
1 large onion, finely chopped
110 g button mushrooms, finely chopped
1 teaspoon soy sauce
1 teaspoon fresh chopped parsley
1 teaspoon fresh thyme
1 380 g tin peeled plum tomatoes
1 clove garlic, crushed
salt and freshly milled black pepper
110 g brown rice
Cook rice in normal way. Drain and chop tomatoes reserving juice for later. Place the onion, garlic and mushrooms in a thick bottomed pan, cover and sweat over a low heat. When soft add tomatoes. Add the rice and seasoning, mix well. Stand the peppers in ovenproof dish, cut the top off each pepper

and take out the seeds and white material. Fill them with the mixture, if it looks dry pour some of the tomato sauce into each pepper. Cover dish and bake in a preheated moderate oven for half and hour, the peppers should be soft.

Leek & potato soup with mussels   serves 4
8 well cleaned & sorted mussels per person
dry cider
Prepare leek and potato soup as before. Put 2 inches of cider in the bottom of a large cooking pot. Add mussels, they will cook in the steam. They are ready when shells open. Discard any unopened mussels. Serve soup in large bowls with mussels on top.

Chicken in the pot   serves 2
2 chicken quarters, skinned
1 onion, 3 leeks, 2 cloves of garlic, chopped
4 carrots, 4 small turnips
1 teaspoon olive oil
glass dry white wine
freshly ground black pepper
leaves from two stalks celery
2 potatoes, cut into quarters
Sweat onion, leek and garlic with the olive oil in a thick bottomed ovenproof dish with the

lid on. Add the chicken, turnips and carrots chopped. Add the white wine and water to almost cover chicken. Then add the potatoes, pepper and celery. Cook in oven 190 C for 1 hour. This is a whole meal in one pot. Add more vegetables if you wish.

Chicken with cider
serves 2

2 boned and skinned chicken breasts or 4 drumsticks
dry cider
8 prunes, pitted
1 large cooking apple
4 oz mushrooms, chopped
1 small onion, finely chopped
1 teaspoon oil, salt and pepper

Put oil in thick bottomed casserole. Sweat onion, then seal chicken by turning it a couple of times in the oil on a high heat. Remove chicken from the pot. Add mushrooms and cook on low heat with lid on until soft. Add chicken, apples and enough cider to just cover. Add prunes. Season to taste. Cook in preheated oven 180 C for 40 minutes with the lid on. Then turn oven to low for 1 hour, to make a thick sauce. Serve with peas, brown bread or new potatoes.

Chicken roast

1 medium sized chicken
1 apple
1 lemon
1 onion
gravy powder

Choose a chicken without much fat evident.
It is best to roast chicken with skin intact and
remove later. Cut the apple, lemon and
onion into quarters and stuff into the chicken
Roast chicken on a spit if possible. If not,
roast in preheated oven at 180 C for one hour
or longer if large chicken. Make gravy with
gravy powder and not fat from chicken. Eat
with peas, new potatoes rolled in low fat,
plain yoghurt and finely chopped fresh parsley. Try carrots with a little powdered
ginger instead of butter.

Grilled fish

Almost any fish can be grilled, but only small
fish are suitable for grilling whole. Plaice,
whiting, sole, trout and herring are good
examples. You need to score or slash the skin
of the fish diagonally, this stops the skin from
splitting and allows the heat to penetrate.
Fresh sardines are good cooked on the barbecue. Larger fish are best grilled as steaks or

cutlets. The surface then needs to be brushed very lightly with melted butter or brushed with low fat milk and rolled in flour to get a light covering. Do not add salt before grilling fish, this makes the fish dry out. Make your own sauces for the fish from tomatoes, shallots and fresh herbs. Do not smother the fish in butter or cream sauces.

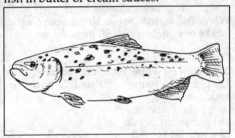

Poached salmon

You can use this method to cook a whole salmon, salmon trout, steaks or fillets. You need enough liquid to barely cover the fish, a container with a lid or enough tin foil to make a loose sealed packet around the fish. A good poaching liquid is half dry white wine, half water with a pinch of dried tarragon. Alternatively you can make a court bouillon.

Use half a pint water, half a bottle dry white wine, bay leaf, 10 peppercorns, blade mace, 2 tablespoons white wine vinegar, half a teaspoon dried tarragon or a tablespoon fresh chervil, one onion, 2 carrots finely sliced Simmer together for half an hour. You can poach on top or in the oven. If on top make sure the liquid does not boil but only simmers. The oven should be set at 180 C. Whole fish up to 6 lb cook 10 mins per pound, steaks or cutlets for 10-20 minutes.

Fisherman's pie
serves 4

225 g skinned white fish fillets, cod or whiting
225 g skinned smoked fish fillets, cod or haddock
50 g frozen peas
450 g mashed potato
25 g low fat spread
25 g plain flour
250 ml semi skimmed milk

Put the milk into a saucepan and add the flour and low fat spread. Slowly bring the sauce to a boil and whisk by hand until sauce thickens. Add salt, pepper and pinch of nutmeg. Preheat the oven to 190 C. Cut the fish into small cubes and mix with peas. Place in an ovenproof dish leaving room for the potato on top. Pour white sauce over the fish, spread mashed potato evenly on top. The potato should cover to the edge of dish to seal moisture in the pie. Bake for 40-45 minutes until the potato is golden brown.

Chill con carne
serves 4

450 g lean minced beef
1 350 g tin peeled plum tomatoes
1 large onion, finely chopped
1 tin red kidney beans, juice drained
2 cloves garlic, finely chopped
2-3 generous teaspoons chilli powder
2 tablespoons tomato puree
half teaspoon dried oregano
half teaspoon dried thyme
2 bayleaves, cayenne pepper, salt
1 beef stock cube in 250 ml water

If you substitute the mince for soya mince and use 2 teaspoons of yeast extract or a vegetable stock cube this can be served as a vegetarian meal. Seal the mince in a heavy frying pan, get the pan very hot, add enough mince to cover bottom of pan. Do not stir or turn mince until it has cooked on one side. When both sides are brown drain off the fat squeezing the mince against the pan with a spatula to drain as much fat as possible.

Cook the meat in several batches. When all ready place in large pan with all the other ingredients. Vary the seasoning to suit your taste. Remember it gets spicier as it cooks. Simmer for 45 mins or longer to thicken sauce. Serve with rice and/or green salad.

Frank's shepherd's pie
serves 4

Courtesy of Frank Wintle, author

The pie has evolved over the years and yours should too. You like sweetcorn? Well then add some sweetcorn. Vary the quantities too, if you feel like it. Anyway this is what I use for four people.

1½lbs the very best minced beef you can get
5 or 6 medium sized potatoes
1 onion, 1 clove of garlic
1 small bag of frozen petit pois
6 cardamoms
pinch thyme, coriander & cumin
6 juniper berries
1 teaspoon olive oil

Peel the potatoes, chop onion and garlic into small pieces, take the seeds from the cardamoms, throw the husks away. Cook the potatoes and juniper berries in lightly salted water for 20 minutes. Cook the peas and put to one side. Heat a heavy frying pan with just enough oil to smear the surface. Take a few cardamom seeds and the other herbs and spices and put them in the hot oil for a minute. Add the garlic and meat. Cook, stirring until the meat is browned all over. Then tip pan to one side and pour off fat. With a slotted spoon transfer it to an ovenproof dish.

Repeat this performance with meat, herbs, spices, onion and garlic until all the mince is in the pie dish. This is the crucial part of the operation. Don't try to fry all your mince in one go. Mix peas in with the meat mixture. Mash the potatoes and spread them on top. At this point you can pause, walk the dog, do the crossword or cast your vote. This dish can be made a day before, which is why it is ideal dinner party fare. To cook, preheat oven to 200 C cook for 45-60 minutes. Serve with a salad, enjoy and improvise.

Hamburger
serves 4

450 g very lean minced beef
1 onion, very finely chopped
1 tablespoon tomato puree
2 tablespoons wholemeal breadcrumbs
1 clove garlic, crushed
freshly milled black pepper

1 egg

Mix everything together and leave for an hour. Pat the meat into shape and cook under a hot grill or on the barbecue. Serve in a wholemeal bun with plenty of coleslaw, made from white cabbage and grated carrot in low fat yoghurt, a squeeze of lemon juice and freshly milled black pepper.

Oranges with crispy toffee

One and a half oranges per person
Enough granulated white sugar to cover the base of a thick bottomed pan
2 teaspoons Poire or Grand Marnier

Remove peel and white pith from oranges. Slice them in very thin rounds. You do need a very thick bottomed pan. Cover base of pan with about 1 cm of sugar, shake gently to get an even covering. Put the pan over lowest heat possible until sugar melts. Do not stir. If one spot melts before the rest turn the pan around. Arrange orange slices singly on a large plate. When the sugar has melted quickly dribble it over the oranges in a criss cross pattern. Prepare the oranges early, but leave the toffee until the last minute or it will go soft. Sprinkle liqueur over just before serving.

Hot pears with blueberries

serves 4

4 large pears, peeled
50 cl red wine
1 cinammon stick
1 tin blueberries in syrup

You can cut pears in half or leave them whole depending on the size of your ovenproof dish.   Add the blueberries and syrup, the wine and cinammon stick, bring to the boil and leave to simmer for 15 mins. Sweeten to taste if necessary. Put dish in preheated oven 200 C.   Cook for 1 hour basting every 15 mins.

Apricot & cherry flan

serves 4

1 medium ready made flan case
Enough low fat yoghurt or low fat creme fraiche (or a mixture of the two) to evenly cover the base of the flan
Tinned apricot halves in fruit juice, or dried apricots soaked overnight
Tinned stoned, black cherries, in juice

Spread yoghurt or creme fraiche over base of flan case, drain juice from tins of fruit and put to one side. Arrange the fruit over the flan. Mix the juice with a little liqueur and pour into a deepish dish. Place the flan on top. The juice is absorbed by the base of the flan.

Green fruit salad

serves 4

1 sweet green melon
2 kiwi fruit
Medium bunch green grapes, peeled
If you have an instrument for making melon balls use this, if not make chunks with a teaspoon.   Peel and slice the kiwi fruit in rounds and mix all together with the grapes. Add a squeeze of lemon juice and some liqueur if you like!

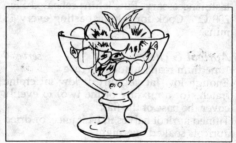

Baked bananas with brown sugar

1 banana per person
1 tablespoon lemon juice per banana
2 teaspoons rum or kirsch per banana
2 teaspoons soft brown sugar per banana
Custard powder and skimmed milk or very

low fat creme fraiche

Cut the bananas longways and lay in an ovenproof dish, pour the lemon juice and rum over bananas and bake in an oven preheated to 180 C. Bake for 15 minutes. Sprinkle brown sugar over them and put under the grill for 5 minutes. The sugar will caramelise. Serve plain, with custard or creme fraiche.

Baked apple

1 large eating apple i.e. Cox's orange or 1 Bramley cooking apple per person
Sultanas, dried currants and mixed peel
1 teaspoon soft brown sugar per apple
fresh squeezed orange juice
orange flower water (optional)

Wash and core apples. Score through skin around the middle of apple. Mix the dried fruit and mixed peel with some brown sugar. Stuff apples with mixture and place in ovenproof dish. Sprinkle rest of sugar over apples and pour the orange juice and flower water around the apples. Bake in a preheated oven 220 C for 25 mins. Do not let juice dry out, add more if necessary. Serve on their own or with very low fat creme fraiche.

Low fat rice pudding

serves 4

1 pint skimmed milk
1 tablespoon short grain pudding rice
artificial sweetener to taste
1 vanilla pod or few drops essence
1 tablespoon sultanas

Soak the rice in the milk for half an hour. Then bring to the boil with sweetener, reduce heat and simmer for 3 minutes. Add sultanas and vanilla or nutmeg. Place mixture in ovenproof dish. Bake in preheated oven 160 C for 2 hours.

Tropical fruit salad

serves 6

1 pineapple, 2 passion fruit
2 large oranges peeled and pithed
1 mango, 2 apples peeled and diced
Seedless grapes or pitted grapes
Juice of one orange and half a lemon

This makes a lot of fruit salad and it will keep until the next day. The lemon juice stops the fruit going brown. Ripe mango and pineapple will make it sweet. Serve with very low fat creme fraiche or nothing at all.

Ice cream

serves 6

fresh or frozen blackberries or raspberries
very low fat creme fraiche (*half weight of fruit*)

2 tablespoons sugar per lb fruit
2 tablespoons water per lb fruit
artificial sweetener if you need it
Cook the fruit in water and sugar until soft,
let mixture cool and liquidise long enough to
mash up fruit but not lose the texture. Add
creme fraiche (*you can use half low fat creme
fraiche and half very low fat plain yoghurt*).
Freeze this mixture (*it will freeze in ice making
compartment*). Let ice cream soften a bit in
fridge for about half an hour before serving.
Eat no more than two scoops per meal!

Mango & passion fruit sorbet   serves 4

2 ripe mangos and 1 passion fruit
1 tablespoon sugar, 2 tablespoons water
Slowly dissolve sugar and water on low heat
to make a syrup. Cool. Liquidise the mango
pulp and inside of passion fruit. Freeze.
After 2 hours check the sorbet. If crystallised
take it out and stir then refreeze. No more
than two scoops per meal!

Raspberry sorbet   serves 4

300 g fresh, frozen or tinned raspberries
100 g castor sugar
half pint water, or syrup from the tin
2 egg whites

For fresh or frozen fruit heat sugar and water to make a syrup. Cool and put aside. Simmer fresh or frozen fruit with a tablespoon of water until soft. Cool, put fruit and syrup in blender. If using tinned put contents straight into blender. Blend and freeze until firm. Beat egg whites until stiff then fold in fruit mixture. Freeze once more until firm. 2 scoop limit again.

Tania's pavlova
serves 8

3 egg whites
6 oz castor sugar
1 level teaspoon cornflour
1 level teaspoon vinegar
Vanilla essence, pinch of salt
Very low fat creme fraiche
2 bananas, 2 passion fruit
1 tin of guava halves

Beat egg whites until stiff and standing in peaks, add the salt and beat in half sugar. Fold in rest of sugar and cornflour. Add one level teaspoon of vinegar and few drops of vanilla essence. Put greaseproof paper on a baking tray and lightly grease. Spoon mixture into middle of paper and spread out evenly making a flat pancake about 3 cm thick. Cook in preheated oven 120 C for 60-

90 minutes then turn oven off and let meringue cool in oven. Just before serving spread creme fraiche over top of meringue base while on serving dish. Arrange slices of banana tossed in lemon juice and the cut up guavas on top. Spoon passion fruit over the other fruits.

Exercises

A most important part of your hip and thigh programme – be sure to make time for these key exercises, aimed at those trouble spots; chins, tummies, hips and thighs. Try to do the exercises in this order, first thing in the morning for 30 days then continue on at least alternate days or four times a week to maintain and continue to improve your new shape. If you find the exercises too easy, do more repetitions. They have all been recommended by physiotherapists or osteopaths. If you experience any pain while doing any of the exercises you should omit them from your programme. Anyone with a history of back or joint pain should always consult their GP or osteopath before undertaking a new exercise programme.

1. Morning stretch

Sit up straight on the edge of your bed when you first wake up. Holding your hands together stretch your arms up towards the ceiling, continue stretching for 10 seconds.

2. Inner thighs

Sit on the edge of your bed or upright chair with your knees bent hip width apart. Push your knees outwards with the palms of your opposite hands while trying to move your knees in. Hold for a few seconds, relax and repeat 10 times.

3. To tighten sagging chins

Looking in the mirror, push you chin as far forward as you can bringing you lower lip up over your top lip at the same time. Relax and repeat ten times. I heard on the radio that Princess Diana uses this exercise as part of her morning routine.

4. For chins and bustline

Clench your teeth and push the corners of your mouth down while pulling your chin up. You should feel the sheet of muscle fibres over you chest and neck tightening. Relax and repeat 10 times.

5. Bust firming

Standing in front of a mirror hold your arms out in front of you at shoulder height. Grasp your forearms with the opposite hands. Keeping your arms at shoulder height and your hands grasped tightly, try and push the bones of your wrists towards your elbows. Relax and repeat twenty times. You should see your breasts and upper chest muscles move up as you are doing this.

6. Upper arms

Standing straight with feet hip width apart, hold your arms straight out to the sides, shoulder height, with palms facing forwards. Clench your fists and bend your elbows so your fists are level with your ears. With your fists clenched all the time push them forwards and down, keeping you elbows at shoulder height – then return slowly to starting position, fists still clenched. Alternate arms and repeat the exercise 20 times each side. This exercise may be hard to do at first, if so start with ten repetitions and work up to 20.

7. Posture

You will never feel in good shape if your

posture is bad. Stand tall and push your shoulders back and your chin forward. Strengthening your stomach muscles helps your posture enormously. Stand in front of the washbasin about 12 inches away. Keeping your back straight bend your knees slightly. Clench your buttocks and tummy muscles and push your bottom forwards. Hold this position for a few seconds then relax muscles and let bottom go back gently. Repeat 10 times.

8. More posture
Lie on the floor hands palms down at your sides, knees bent, feet hip width apart. Tighten tummy muscles and push lower back into the floor as hard as you can. Relax and repeat 10 times.

9. Buttocks
Lying in the same position tighten tummy muscles again and keeping waist on the floor lift hips by contracting your buttocks. Hold for a few seconds. Relax and repeat 10 times.

10. Even more posture
Roll onto your tummy and lie with your toes pointed behind you, hands flat on the floor

just under your shoulders. Push your head and chest upwards keeping your hips on the floor. Then bend your head back. Hold for a few seconds relax and repeat 10 times.

11. For hips and thighs

Kneel up on all fours, keeping your knees and hands hip width apart. Lift your left leg still bent at the knee out to the side. Do not lean on the opposite hand but keep weight evenly distributed. Repeat with alternate legs 10 times.

12. Stomach, hips and thighs

Kneel straight up keeping knees hip width apart and tighten your tummy muscles. Hold your arms out at shoulder height with palms facing upwards. Gently lean backwards to make a 'Z' shape – your back must stay straight. Go back to the upright position having held the 'Z' for a few seconds. Repeat 10 times.

Finish your exercises by standing up straight, feet hip width apart, buttocks clenched, tummy muscles tightened and stretching up to the ceiling. Hold for ten seconds then relax and shake arms and legs loosely.

Maintenance programme

Now you have read the diet information and practised the menus by following the diet for one month, you are in a position to adjust your eating habits without too much frustration. Reduce your fat intake and select the exercises you feel are benefiting you most. Your maintenance plan can be as simple or as complicated as you choose. You may cut out certain foods completely, reduce your intake of some and eat more of others. You may like to continue planning menus a week ahead to balance your diet. Eat a larger breakfast and increase the size of portions but try not to increase your daily intake of fat. Keep doing some exercises. It is your maintenance programme – you design it so that you know you will enjoy it. You have all the information you need right here and the chance to be a fitter, shapelier person right now.

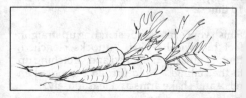

	Fat per 100g		Fibre per 100g
	oz	100g	oz	100g
Apple, baked in skin	0	0	1	2
Apricot, dried	0	0	7	24
Avocado pear	6	22	1	2
Bacon rashers, grilled	5	19	0	0
Beans baked in tomato sauce	0	1	2	7
Beef, corned	3	12	0	0
Beef, roast sirloin	6	21	0	0
Beef steak rump, grilled	2	6	0	0
Beefburgers, low fat	4	13	0	0
Bran flakes	1	2	4	15
Bread, brown	1	2	1	5
Camembert	7	24	0	0
Cheese biscuits	8	30	0	0
Cheshire cheese	9	31	0	0
Chicken stock cubes	6	21	0	0
Chips, potato	3	10	0	0
Chocolate, plain	8	24	0	0
Chocolate digestive biscuits	8	25	1	3
Christmas pudding	3	12	1	2
Cocktail gherkins	0	0	0	0
Cream, single	5	19	0	0
Cream, whipping	11	39	0	0
Cream of chicken soup	1	4	0	0
Crisps potato	10	37	3	12
Crispbread, wheat	2	8	1	5

	Fat per 100g		Fibre per 100g	
---	oz	100g	oz	100g
Croissants	7	24	0	0
Custard, egg	2	6	0	0
Custard, instant	0	1	0	0
Dover sole, fresh	0	1	0	0
Duck, roast meat fat, skin	8	30	0	0
Eggs, fried	6	20	0	0
Fish pie	2	6	0	0
Fishfingers, fried	4	13	0	0
Frankfurters	7	25	0	0
French salad dressing	16	55	0	0
Fromage frais, very low fat	0	0	0	0
Fruit salad, tinned	0	0	0	0
Ginger nuts	4	15	1	2
Gouda cheese	7	23	0	0
Haddock fillets, fresh	0	1	0	0
Ice cream chocolate	6	20	0	0
Kidney beans, red tinned	0	1	3	9
Lamb chops, grilled	8	30	0	0
Lamb's kidney	2	6	0	0
Lemon sole fillets, fresh	0	1	0	0
Minestrone, tinned	0	1	0	0
Moussaka	4	13	0	0
Mustard, English	3	10	0	0
Mustard, French	1	4	0	0
Nice biscuits	5	16	0	0

	oz	Fat per 100g	oz	Fibre per 100g
Omelette, plain	5	16	0	0
Oysters, raw	0	1	0	0
Pancakes	5	16	0	1
Pasty, Cornish	6	20	0	0
Pastry, flaky cooked	12	41	1	2
Pastry, shortcrust	9	32	1	2
Peanut butter	14	51	2	8
Pheasant, roast	3	9	0	0
Pilchards in sauce	2	5	0	0
Plaice fillet, fresh	0	2	0	0
Polony sausage	6	21	0	0
Pork chop, grilled	7	25	0	0
Pork, roast leg	6	20	0	0
Pork, luncheon meat	7	25	1	2
Pork pate & mushrooms	9	32	0	0
Pork pie, Melton	8	29	0	0
Pork sausage, grilled	7	25	0	0
Potato, baked in jacket	0	0	1	3
Prawns, fresh	0	1	0	0
Processed cheese	8	30	0	0
Profiterôles	8	28	0	0
Rabbit, stewed	2	10	0	0
Ratatouille	1	3	0	1
Salami, average	13	45	0	0
Salmon, smoked Scottish	3	10	0	0

		Fat per		Fibre per
	oz	100g	oz	100g
Sardines, tinned in oil	8	28	0	0
Sardines in tomato sauce	3	12	0	0
Scampi, fried, breadcrumb	5	18	0	0
Scones	4	15	1	2
Scotch egg	6	20	0	0
Smoked mackerel, fresh	4	15	0	0
Smoked salmon, fresh	3	10	0	0
Smoked trout	6	22	0	0
Sole, dover fresh	0	1	0	0
Soufflé cheese	5	20	0	0
Southern stir fry	0	1	1	4
Spaghetti, boiled	0	0	0	2
Sponge cake, with fat	5	20	0	1
Sponge flan case	1	3	0	0
Steak & kidney pie	4	15	0	0
Stilton cheese	11	40	0	0
Sugar puffs	0	1	2	6
Sultanas, dried	0	0	2	7
Tagliatelle, cooked	0	0	0	2
Taramasalata	12	41	0	0
Thousand Island dressing	7	25	0	0
Tomato ketchup, average	0	1	0	0
Tuna fish in oil	5	17	0	0
Weetabix/Weetaflakes	1	3	4	13
White fish fillets, frozen	0	1	0	0
Yorkshire pudding	3	10	0	1